The information presented herein represents the views of the author as of the date of publication. This book is presented for informational purposes only. Due to the rate at which conditions change, the author reserves the right to alter and update his opinions at any time. While every attempt has been made to verify the information in this book, the author does not assume any responsibility for errors, inaccuracies, or omissions.

This book is not intended as a substitute for the medical advice of physicians. The reader should regularly consult a physician in matters relating to his/her health and particularly with respect to any symptoms that may require diagnosis or medical attention.

Contents

Introduction

My name is Jim Twomey. I am fifty-five years old. I am extremely fortunate to be free of pain, and I enjoy my life.

I'm a pain relief specialist. For the last seventeen years, I have been committed to making a difference for others. I've had the dream of healing people from their afflictions. For the last thirteen years I've been helping people with emotional problems. This includes relieving anxiety and depression, and other challenges. I help people experience joy and peace. I help them break through and get to a place of contentment and satisfaction, even happiness. We use laughter, breathing exercises, meditation, going into nature, presence, and more. It's very fulfilling and I love doing it.

I noticed that many of my clients also had physical pain. I thought, "How can I reduce people's physical pain? How can I help people break through their discomfort and get to a better place?" For years I had been healing back pain, joint pain, and more, for both myself and my family. I had been using low-level laser, supplements, and relaxing exercises to help reduce pain and inflammation. Since I started practicing pain relief on myself and my family, we have been moving easier and more comfortably. We have been getting fast results in a healthy way. No side effects. And I have not been toxifying or drugging myself or my family, or creating scar tissue for us.

I thought, "I can do this for others." So now I'm also healing people from physical pain. I am using a low-level laser, supplements, relaxing exercises, and more to help reduce people's physical pain and heal them. I also suggest foods and drinks to either consume or avoid, which can help reduce pain and inflammation.

People are helped from head to toe. Neck, shoulders, elbows, wrists, hands, upper back, mid back, lower back, hips, knees, ankles, feet, and toes are healed. Depression, anxiety, traumatic brain injury, concussions, tinnitus, frozen shoulder, stenosis, restless leg, osteoarthritis, and more have been helped. Tendinitis has been cured. Low-level laser regenerates all tissue: muscle, tendon, ligament, cartilage, bone, and brain. Aches are reduced. I support people in their overall health. People feel relaxed. Low-level laser is FDA approved for pain relief, inflammation reduction, and increased blood circulation. The first session is free and all treatment is guaranteed. I can even come to your home. People get back to walking, dancing, and golfing. They get back to leading their lives the way they want to live them. I help people transform their lives.

This book is for people who have physical pain and who want to be more comfortable. This book is especially for those people who sincerely believe they need to take painkilling drugs for the rest of their lives. I agree that pharmaceuticals can have their place in a thoughtful treatment plan, and for some people they can be very effective. But they should always be used with the lowest dose possible and in conjunction with the many available non-invasive and safe techniques that are presented in this book. My hope is that if you are suffering from chronic pain, or even "normal" aches and pains, and you are taking pain medication, that you consult with your prescribing physician and explore how you can reduce—and even put aside—your painkilling drugs.

My goal—and the goal of this book—is to show you a healthy way you can reduce your pain and heal both your mind and your body.

That's why we're here today, so let's get started!

Chapter 1: The Miracle of Low-Level Laser Therapy

Let's begin with a conversation with my friend and colleague Doug about an amazing therapy that I've been using to relieve pain. For many of my clients, low-level laser therapy has lifted their burden of pain and given them a sense of freedom they hadn't felt in a long time. Many say the healing power of the low-level laser is almost miraculous. It may seem that way, but in fact—as we'll learn in the pages ahead—it's power to relieve pain is based on real science.

Doug: What is a fast and healthy way to get pain relief and healing?

Jim: I recommend low-level laser therapy as the fast way to relieve pain and get healing. A laser is a device that emits electromagnetic radiation in the optical region. It produces a beam. A laser is a tool. It is a light amplifier. The light can penetrate up to nine inches deep. Much of the healing using infrared light is in the one- to three-inch deep area.

Doug: I thought surgical lasers were used to cut tissues, not heal them.

Jim: Cool laser therapy is low-intensity laser therapy, or laser therapy that uses low levels of light to stimulate healing. Cold laser therapy is sometimes called low-level laser therapy (LLLT), low-power laser therapy (LPLT), or soft laser. You may also hear it referred to as therapeutic laser, biostimulation, or photobiomodulation. Unlike surgical or aesthetic lasers, it does not cause your tissues to heat up. When you direct the beam onto the skin, there's no sensation of heat.

Laser power is measured in milliwatts and watts. LLLT uses red beam or near infrared nonthermal lasers with a wavelength between 600 and 1000 nanometers and from five to 1,000 milliwatts. In contrast, lasers used for surgery typically use 300 watts. That's a big difference!

Doug: Who invented the therapeutic use of nonthermal or cool lasers?

Jim: Hungarian physician and surgeon Endre Mester is credited with the discovery of the biological effects of low-level lasers. A few years after the 1960 invention of the ruby laser and the 1961 invention of the helium–neon (HeNe) laser, which are both "hot" lasers, Mester experimented with a standard ruby laser light to try to replicate an experiment that showed that such hot lasers could reduce tumors in mice. During his experiments, he accidentally discovered that the laser could regrow hair on the mice. He then discovered the laser he was using was faulty and wasn't as powerful as he thought. While the low-level laser failed to affect the tumors, he noticed that where he had shaved the mice in order to do the experiments, the hair grew back faster in those places where he had treated with the laser, compared with the placebos.

He published his findings in 1967. He went on to show that low-level HeNe light could accelerate wound healing in mice. In 1971, he began treating patients with non-healing skin ulcers while using low intensity laser irradiation. In 1974 he founded the Laser Research Center at the Semmelweis Medical University in Budapest, and continued working there until he died in 1984. His two sons, Adam Mester, M.D., a radiologist, and Andrew Mester, M.D., an otolaryngologist, continued his work and brought it to the United States.

Doug: So there's a solid scientific basis for the effectiveness of low-level laser to heal!

Jim: Absolutely. And there have been dozens of scientific research studies that have confirmed it, which I'll talk about in the pages ahead.

How the Laser Works

Doug: How does low-level laser therapy work?

Jim: Low-level light is applied directly to the painful area—joint, muscle, bone, nerve, skin, brain. The tissue then absorbs the light, which triggers a biological or chemical reaction to red and near infrared light. Damaged cells have a physiological reaction that helps promote their regeneration.

Depending on the purpose of the treatment, differing wavelengths and outputs may be used. Typically, wavelengths between 600 and 700 nanometers (nm) are used to treat superficial tissue. Longer wavelengths between 780 and 950 nm are used for deeper penetration.

Doug: Does the client feel any pain from the laser?

Jim: Absolutely not! During the procedure, the client feels the device against his or her skin, but it creates no heat, sound, or vibration. It's completely noninvasive and painless. Most of the time, one treatment will take only a few minutes.

Doug: It affects the tissues?

Jim: It will regenerate tissue, muscles, ligaments, tendons, cartilage, bone, and the brain.

Doug: What does low-level laser therapy involve?

Jim: It's simple. You shine the light on the area of pain. We are exposing the cells or tissue to low levels of red and near-infrared light. Red and infrared light stimulates, heals, regenerates and protects tissue that has either been injured, is degenerating, or else is at risk of dying.

Doug: What does low-level therapy do to cells?

Jim: It heals, energizes, regenerates, and increases the oxygen to the cells. Laser puts energy into the cells.

Doug: Can the low-level laser treatment burn us?

Jim: No. It is a cool laser, not a hot laser. Hot lasers can damage cells. Cool lasers heal cells.

Doug: How is the laser used?

Jim: We shine the light on the area of pain and inflammation. It's actually a bit more complicated than that, but that's the simple way to talk about it. So if there's an injury to, let's say, somebody's bicep, I laser the area of pain in the bicep. I would treat the painful area coming from four different places on the upper arm. Ten seconds to one minute per area.

Doug: Is the healing permanent?

Jim: That depends on the person. They get pain relief and healing. But if they go out and do an arduous workout, they can reinjure the area. Remember, we're talking about living tissue. It's constantly changing and renewing itself. The human body's ability to replace worn out cells with new ones is key to our long lifespan. There are a few cells we keep all our lives, like the ones in the visual cortex, but most cells in your body wear out and get replaced. Each type of cell has its own lifespan. For example, skin cells are known to live about 14 days. Muscle cells can live up to 15 years. The cells lining your gut last about five days. And they're all subject to damage from disease, injury, or just normal wear and tear. The low-level laser is very effective at relieving pain at the moment of treatment, and then for as long as conditions don't change. And for many people, this lifting of their pain is like a dream come true. Some of my clients call it a miracle. But it's not a miracle—it's science.

Doug: Does it hurt?

Jim: No. It's relaxing. Some people even feel their pain reducing during the treatment. Others find the treatment soothing. One of my patients loves it; she's like, "Laser me here, laser me there." Because it's non-invasive and harmless, I accommodate her, as long as we get the primary job done.

Doug: Has a low-level laser hurt anyone's eyes?

Jim: To my knowledge, nobody has suffered eye damage from a low-level laser. I would never recommend looking directly into it, because it's like any other bright light. During treatment we're very careful not to shine it into the client's eyes. The session is supposed to be soothing, not like you're being interrogated!

The International Electrotechnical Commission (IEC) has categorized lasers by class. The class reflects the power of the laser and how "hot" it is—meaning whether or not it will heat your tissues. These are the four basic classes and their relative eye safety. Remember, the following comments relate *only to eye safety*. Lasers of all classes are used in therapeutic settings, even powerful Class 4 lasers.

Class 1: This class is eye-safe under all operating conditions.

Class 1M: This class is safe for viewing directly with the naked eye, but may be hazardous to view with the aid of optical instruments that would magnify the beam, such as binoculars or telescopes. Radiation in classes 1 and 1M can be visible, invisible, or both.

Class 2: These are visible lasers. This class is safe for accidental viewing under all operating conditions. However, it may not be safe for a person who, by overcoming their natural aversion response to the very bright light, deliberately stares into the laser beam for longer than 0.25 seconds.

Class 2M: These are visible lasers. This class is safe for accidental viewing with the naked eye, as long as the natural aversion response is not overcome as with Class 2, but may be hazardous (even for accidental viewing) when viewed with the aid of optical instruments, as with class 1M.

Light energy in classes 2 and 2M is visible, but can also contain an invisible element, subject to certain conditions.

Class 3R: Light energy in this class is considered low risk when used professionally.

Class 3B: Light energy in this class is significant and should be handled by a professional with care. For a continuous wave laser, the maximum output into the eye must not exceed 500mW. While the light energy can be a hazard to the eye, viewing of the diffuse reflection is safe. In my practice, I use a Class 3B pulse laser. Because I'm a trained professional, it is absolutely safe.

Class 4: This is the highest class of laser light energy. Viewing of the diffuse reflection may be damaging. Class 4 lasers for phototherapy have been on the market for years but have been approved strictly for surgical applications, such as general surgery and tissue ablation for port wine stains, and spider veins.

Doug: How often does a person need a laser treatment?

Jim: It depends. One to six times can help relieve pain and heal. Some people can use a monthly treatment and some weekly. When someone has an injury, they can maybe use three times a week in the beginning. I have cured a woman with tendinitis. For most people, they get pain relief and healing. They can get active again and do what they want.

Doug: What is low-level laser F.D.A. approved for?

Jim: The Food and Drug Administration has approved it for pain reduction, inflammation reduction, and increased blood flow.

Doug: What are the side effects of low-level laser treatment?

Jim: None, zero. It's very exciting that it relieves pain and there are no side effects. The worst thing that can happen is that nothing happens.

Doug: Does low-level laser helps in healing?

Jim: Yes. It heals muscles, ligament, cartilage, bone, and brain tissue. It regenerates and energizes. There's tissue oxygenation and reduced swelling, it helps you feel more comfortable, and it's relaxing. Most people have pain relief after the first treatment. And when I do my first treatment for people, it is free—they have nothing to lose but their pain!

Doug: What can you help?

Jim: Many things. I can help people recover from surgery, osteoarthritis, fibromyalgia, and plantar fasciitis. I help people head to toe: head, neck, shoulders, elbows, wrists, fingers, back, hips, knees, ankles, feet, and toes. And it's also very exciting that it heals the brain.

Doug: Can you help back pain?

Jim: Yes. I help people with their upper back, middle back, and lower back. It is relaxing and the treatment takes less than five minutes.

Doug: Can you help relieve joint pain?

Jim: Yes. I help shoulders, elbows, wrists, fingers, knees, ankles, and toes.

Doug: Can you help people recover from surgery?

Jim: Laser is great at helping people heal from surgery. It reduces the pain, inflammation, redness, and swelling. I have helped people after back and ankle surgeries.

Doug: Can you help people recover from injuries?

Jim: Yes. I help people with strains and sprains, pulls, and tears. I help rotator cuff injuries. Head to toe. One of my clients had a knee injury. I helped to recover him so that he could get back to running. I help people get back to walking, dancing, golfing, working out, and going to the gym.

Doug: Can osteoarthritis be helped?

Jim: Low-level laser can help osteoarthritis. I have helped people with knee osteoarthritis. People can expect pain relief. They can also expect an increased range of movement and reduced swelling.

Doug: What about an auto accident?

Jim: Yes, I can help people with such injuries. Help reduce the pain, increase blood circulation to that area, and heal them.

Doug: How about falls?

Jim: Yes, definitely. People fall from different things, but we can heal that. Heal the ligaments and tendons. And I'm not going to say it is 100 percent. If you have somebody who had a serious car accident, I can help to heal, but I can't say they're going to be perfect again. But I can help reduce the pain and make them feel better.

Doug: Can you help fibromyalgia?

Jim: Laser regenerates damaged muscle and nerves. Laser can reduce the pain from fibromyalgia. And there can be slow and steady improvement.

Doug: Can laser help shingles (herpes zoster)?

Jim: There will be a decrease in pain using laser followed by the disappearance of the lesions. A treatment plan can be treatments twice weekly for three weeks is appropriate for acute cases, followed by once per week after there has been a significant decrease in pain.

Doug: Can you help tinnitus?

Jim: Laser can be very effective with tinnitus. Tinnitus can be cured. My first client's tinnitus is down 90% after eight treatments! Sometimes he can't even hear it.

Doug: Can you reduce wrinkles?

Jim: Yes, wrinkles can be lessened. You can expect to look ten years younger. Improvement is noticeable after the first treatment.

Doug: Can carpal tunnel syndrome be cured?

Jim: Yes. Laser is a powerful healer of carpal tunnel. Decreased pain and increased function and strength can be expected.

Doug: What are some untreatable issues you can help?

Jim: Trigger finger can be gotten rid of. Dupuytren's contracture can be improved. (This is a hand deformity that usually develops over years. The condition affects a layer of tissue that lies under the skin of your palm, causing your fingers to curl inwards, like you were holding a baseball.) I have made plantar fasciitis a non-issue for myself. Heel pain can be helped.

Doug: Can you treat every issue that has pain, soreness, or injury?

Jim: No, I can't treat everything. The laser can treat two to three inches deep; it can go up to nine inches deep. So if someone who has an issue, let's say eight inches deep, the laser might not be able to do a lot with that. When I laser somebody's ankle, that treatment also goes to the brain. There's a secondary impact on the brain, which is healing. So, laser can't heal all the kinds of pain. It can do many types of issues, reduce many types of pain, and there are no side effects. Try it, and if it doesn't work, there's no cost.

Doug: So if it goes eight inches into my body with the laser, is it damaging the tissue in-between? You know, that's going to hit everything right?

Jim: The laser is healing for all the tissues. It's healing for blood, and of course muscles, ligaments, tendons, cartilage, bone, and brain tissue. It heals all the tissue.

Doug: How expensive is the laser treatment?

Jim: The first treatment is free. If it's just a few treatments and it is quick, so it could be $97. But if it's an ongoing program, then it's going to be more expensive. So it depends what a person has going on.

Healing the Brain

Doug: Is it true that low-level laser can heal the brain?

Jim: Yes. This is very exciting. Laser regenerates all tissue, reduces inflammation, increases blood flow, improves oxygenation, and helps the brain repair itself. It helps memory and sleep. I helped a client with his sleep. It increases regional cerebral blood flow and improves cognition (executive function and verbal memory). I have helped people with brain damage, depression, concussions, and traumatic brain injury.

Joe had six treatments. He is having musical compositions coming to him now. Full symphonies are coming into his head. That was not happening before the laser. I can help people with their mood. I can help people with ALS, Alzheimer's disease, dementia, encephalitis, Meniere's disease, MLS, Parkinson's disease, post-traumatic stress disorders, and again sleep. Michael Hamblin (Ph.D.), Wellman Center for Photomedicine at Harvard Medical School, is doing a lot of research on healing the brain. There are scientific studies that show it helps depression, strokes, traumatic brain injury, and more. And again, there are no side effects. The treatment is 60 seconds long and relaxing. So that is very exciting to heal people's brains.

The brain suffers from many different disorders that can be classified into three broad groupings: traumatic events (stroke, traumatic brain injury, and global ischemia), degenerative diseases (dementia, Alzheimer's and Parkinson's), and psychiatric disorders (depression, anxiety, post-traumatic stress disorder). There is some evidence that all these seemingly diverse conditions can be beneficially affected by applying light to the head. Low-level laser therapy can also be called photobiomodulation. It increases cerebral blood flow, greater oxygen availability, and oxygen consumption. Laser can be used for cognitive enhancement in healthy people. A scientific study was done on this. The light is applied to the forehead. Laser stimulates brain opioids—endorphins and serotonin. Circulation is increased.

Dr. Michael Hamblin is the expert in this area. A professor at Harvard Medical School, Dr. Hamblin has published nearly three hundred peer-reviewed articles, over 150 conference proceedings, book chapters and international abstracts, and he holds eight patents. He has edited the most recent and comprehensive textbook on photodynamic therapy entitled *Advances in Photodynamic Therapy: Basic, Translational and Clinical*, and he's edited or written dozens more.

As his biography on the website of the Wellman Center for Photomedicine says, "Applications of LLLT to healing and treatment of traumatic brain injury are being studied. Results from these studies have suggested that transcranial near-infrared (NIR) light may have wide applications to a diverse range of brain disorders, including stroke; neurodegenerative diseases such as Alzheimer's and Parkinson's; and psychiatric disorders such as depression, anxiety, PTSD, autism, and addiction." That's great news for people suffering with a disorder of the brain!

Depression and Alzheimer's Disease

Doug: Does laser help depression?

Jim: Yes. I have helped five people with depression. Laser heals the brain. There is a scientific study out of Harvard showing low-level laser helping people with depression. One client has been feeling silly at times. The treatment time is less than 60 seconds. Results are noticeable after three treatments. Prescription drugs for depression are not regarded very highly by the medical profession, perform little better than placebos in different trials, and moreover can also have significant side effects. Low-level laser for depression is a much healthier way to go that drugs for depression.

In 2009, researcher F. Schiffer and others took ten patients with a history of major depression and anxiety (including post-traumatic stress disorder and substance abuse) and applied low-level laser light to their foreheads for four weeks. At the end of the study, six of the ten patients experienced a remission of their depression, and seven of the ten patients experienced a remission of their anxiety. There were no observable side effects. This seems reasonable because several studies have shown that depression is linked to abnormal blood flow in the frontal cortex of the brain, and low-level lasering increases blood flow and circulation.

Doug: Does laser help dementia and Alzheimer's?

Jim: Low-level laser inhibits cell death and slows the progression of dementia and Alzheimer's. A key study was performed by Kazuyoshi Zenba, vice president of Kanagawa Acupuncture Massage Association and Professor Masayuki Inoue, Secretary of JLPLTPA. They wrote in "The Efficacy of 904 nm Laser Therapy for Alzheimer's Diseases" that after the start of low-level laser treatment, the coldness of the hands and legs of patients vanished, and the stiffness of their joints and muscles was also mitigated. For caregivers, it became easier to care for patients. All fifteen patients came to show better understanding of the directions of the care workers. It was suggested by this that low-level laser could be a practical treatment of patients at home. They also stated, "the advance of condition of Alzheimer's diseases has been blocked." That's very good news!

Doug: What about Bell's palsy?

Jim: Laser can help a person feel more comfortable, especially at night, after the first treatment. Science supports this. In 2014, M.S. Alayat and others published their study, "Efficacy of high and low level laser therapy in the treatment of Bell's palsy: a randomized double blind placebo-controlled trial," in which they concluded "both HILT [high intensity laser therapy] and LLLT are effective physical therapy modalities for the recovery of patients with Bell's palsy, with HILT showing a slightly greater improvement than LLLT." Many others have produced the same results.

Doug: Are you the only person in Tucson healing people's brains?

Jim: While I probably am not, I don't know of anyone else doing it. And there are no side effects using a low-level laser. It heals the brain.

Doug: From whom did you learn?

Jim: I have learned a great deal from Dr. Curtis Turchin, an internationally known expert in the field of laser therapy for the treatment of acute and chronic pain. He has used laser treatment for nearly thirty years and serves as director of clinical sciences for Apollo Lasers.

Dr. Turchin is an established leader in the industry, authoring four books and more than twenty journal articles on laser therapy. He's the author of *Light and Laser Therapy: Clinical Procedures*, the best clinical manual available on the use of low level lasers. He lectures at numerous chiropractic colleges and state associations in the US and has taught therapists and doctors in Europe, Japan, Brazil, Canada and Guatemala.

I have also learned from the book *Laser Phototherapy* by Lars Hode and Jan Tuner. It's an invaluable guide to the current literature and a wealth of laser therapy knowledge. The book contains over 900 pages and 2,500 references, and is a thorough update of their 2010 book, *The New Laser Therapy Handbook*. Lars Hode is a physicist, and has specialized in medical laser applications and working with laser therapy since 1983. He is the president and founder of the Swedish Laser-Medical Society 1989. Jan Tuner is a renowned Swedish dentist who has worked with therapeutic lasers for more than thirty years. As a lecturer, he's been invited to several universities and congresses worldwide and was a teacher at the European Master degree in Oral Laser Applications for many years.

Scientific Studies Support Low-Level Laser Therapy

Doug: What proof exists that low-level laser therapy relieves pain?

Jim: There are many scientific studies supporting low-level laser therapy. You can go to the National Institute of Health, US National Library of Medicine, Pubmed.gov website (.ncbi.nlm.nih.gov/PubMed). You can search "low-level laser therapy."

For example, a 2004 study entitled "Low-Level Laser Therapy Facilitates Superficial Wound Healing in Humans: A Triple-Blind, Sham-Controlled Study" concluded, "The LLLT resulted in enhanced healing as measured by wound contraction. The untreated wounds in subjects treated with LLLT contracted more than the wounds in the sham group, so LLLT may produce an indirect healing effect on surrounding tissues. These data indicate that LLLT is an effective modality to facilitate wound contraction of partial-thickness wounds."

In the 2010 study "Anti-Inflammatory Effect of Low-Level Laser and Light-Emitting Diode in Zymosan-Induced Arthritis," researchers concluded, "Irradiation with 685 nm and 830 nm laser wavelengths significantly inhibited edema formation, vascular permeability, and hyperalgesia. Laser irradiation, averaged over the two wavelengths, reduced the vascular permeability by 24%, edema formation by 23%, and articular incapacitation by 59 percent." (Edema is a condition characterized by an excess of watery fluid collecting in the cavities or tissues of the body. Hyperalgesia is an increased sensitivity to pain, which may be caused by damage to nociceptors or peripheral nerves. Lowering either one is good!)

Another study found that low-level laser treatments can help heal damaged nerves. In "New trend in neuroscience: Low-power laser effect on peripheral and central nervous system (basic science, preclinical and clinical studies)," researchers stated, "using LPLI may improve neuronal metabolism, prevent neuronal degeneration, and promote improved spinal cord function and repair," and "LPLI has a 'preventive' and therapeutic effect which can be used in different neurosurgical situations associated with peripheral and central nervous system injuries and disorders."

There are many more scientific studies on Alzheimer's, carpal tunnel, chronic joint disorders, depression, edema, fibromyalgia, knee pain, neck pain, arthritis, traumatic brain injury, TMJ, wound healing, and more.

Doug: What evidence is there that low-level laser helps back pain?

Jim: There was a metadata study done, reviewing many different studies. This is from 2015. The conclusion was that "our findings indicate that low-level laser therapy is an effective method for treating patients with chronic low back pain." I've had a lot of success helping people with their low back pain.

Doug: Does low-level laser therapy reduce joint pain?

Jim: There was a systematic review of joint pain studies in 2012. The conclusion was that the review showed that "laser therapy on the joint reduces pain in patients." And I've helped people with their shoulders, elbows, wrists, fingers, hips, knees, ankles, feet and toes.

Doug: What do the scientific studies show on low-level laser and shoulder tendinopathy?

Jim: For shoulder and laser therapy, there was a review of studies done in 2015. The conclusion was, "This review shows that low-level laser therapy can offer clinically relevant pain relief and initiate a more rapid course of improvement." So, it's healing and regenerating. I have helped people with frozen shoulder and rotation cuff injuries.

Doug: I've even heard about using low-level laser to reduce gingivitis!

Jim: Yes. Gingivitis is a common form of gum disease (periodontal disease) that causes irritation, redness and swelling (inflammation) of your gingiva, the part of your gum around the base of your teeth. In "The Effects of Low Level Laser Irradiation on Gingival Inflammation," researchers reported, "a general conclusion can be drawn that low level laser irradiation (semiconductor, 670 nm) can be used as a successful physical adjuvant method of treatment, which, together with traditional periodontal therapy, leads to better and longer-lasting therapeutic results."

There are literally hundreds more studies that support the therapeutic and healing value of low-level lasers. But the very best evidence comes from the many clients I've treated who find real pain relief and who can now wake up every morning with confidence and a positive attitude. Being free from pain can change your life. It's like going from night to day.

Chapter 2: The Danger of Opioids

Doug: Why shouldn't I use painkilling drugs for more than two weeks to manage the pain from an injury or operation?

Jim: The issue is that many people are dying from becoming addicted to some painkilling drugs, while the low-level laser has zero side effects. Many painkilling drugs are risky to take.

Doug: Why are opioids so dangerous? How do you get addicted?

Jim: They chemically target the brain's reward system and alter it. There's a part of the brain that is activated by both natural rewards such as food and by artificial rewards such as addictive drugs. This part of the brain is called the reward system, and it's vital for human survival. Neuroscientists have been able to pinpoint the exact parts of the brain involved—they include the ventral tegmental area, the nucleus accumbens, and the prefrontal cortex. The problem with opiates—as well as other addictive substances like nicotine and cocaine—is that they don't just have an effect and then wear off, leaving no damage. Opioids actually alter the brain cells—the neurons—so that they can't function normally without more opioids! Continued use of opiates makes the brain rely on the presence of the drug to maintain rewarding feelings and other normal behaviors. The person is no longer able to feel the benefits of natural rewards such as food, water, and even sex, and can't function without the drug present. This is why even the strongest person can become addicted to opioids. They change your brain chemistry and when you stop taking the drugs you can become violently ill.

Doug: How many people die every year from prescription opioids?

Jim: About 32,000 people die each year from prescription opioids. This is from 2015, from the Centers for Disease Control and Prevention (CDC). These are narcotics. Oxycodone, OxyContin are the brand names. Acetaminophen/Oxycodone: Percocet is the brand name. Hydrocodone: Vicodin is the brand name. Morphine, codeine, Oxymorphone, and fentanyl are more. I understand that there's a time and place for narcotics. Death from opioid pain relievers is a modern epidemic.

My mom and dad were each dying from cancer. They took morphine to ease the pain. They needed that at the end of their lives. So there are times to take prescription opioids.

Prescription opioids are risky, especially taking them for more than two weeks. There's a risk of dependence and addiction.

Doug: Who are these people who become addicted?

Jim: I treated a woman whose her husband was a pharmacist who committed suicide at home, and he was addicted to oxycodone. So, I think there are lots of people out there that have an injury; their doctor gave them a narcotic because they're in a lot of pain. And then they stay on the drug, they get addicted, they don't try anything else, and then they get in trouble.

Doug: Why take it?

Jim: People take it because they are in pain. When they take it for two weeks or more, they get into a habit, and if they don't do anything to address the underlying problem; the next thing you know is that they are addicted, and they can't get off it.

Doug: Are these weak people?

Jim: No, they are not. We've had friends who have been on narcotics.

Doug: So it can be anybody?

Jim: Yes. It can be anybody. Absolutely.

Other Drugs Are Dangerous Too

Doug: How many people die yearly from non-steroidal anti-inflammatory drugs (NSAIDS)?

Jim: About 15,000 people per year die from non-steroidal anti-inflammatory drugs. This is according to Stanford's Dr. Sean Mackey. He's a past president of the American Academy of Pain Medicine, and has built Stanford's pain center into one of the nation's most comprehensive and well-funded pain research operations. Aspirin, Celebrex, Ibuprofen (Motrin, Advil), Aleve and more are examples.

Doug: How many people die from prescription opioids and non-steroidal anti-inflammatory drugs per year?

Jim: It's about 47,000 people a year die from the prescriptions opioids and non-steroidal anti-inflammatory drugs. That is 47,000 dead Americans per year. This is insane! These painkilling drugs are killers. They are dangerous. There are alternatives. Well, that's a lot of people who are dying, and to me, we have to look for what are other alternatives for people to get pain relief.

Doug: What are the side effects of prescription opioids and non-steroidal anti-inflammatory drugs?

Jim: For prescription opioids, side effects some people have are constipation, nausea, vomiting, and drowsiness. For the non-steroidal anti-inflammatory drugs, some people have nausea, vomiting, diarrhea, constipation, decreased appetite, rash, dizziness, headaches, and drowsiness. So these drugs are unhealthy. They screw up your gastrointestinal tract. The drugs are toxic, and they're risky and dangerous. Drugs are not a healthy way to deal with pain. I understand that drugs are an easy way to relieve pain. They don't resolve the underlying issue. Drugs don't heal tissue. They damage the body, especially over the long term.

The wrong way to handle pain is to go on a narcotic and then do nothing else to relieve your pain and heal. That is a recipe for addiction and is dangerous.

Doug: Are measures now being taken to control the distribution of opioids helping?

Jim: Frankly, no, because there are too many addicts who need to be weaned off narcotics. Experts have noted that, as opioid restrictions tighten, the traditional medical system and insurance industry have not done enough to support opioid-withdrawal efforts, show more physicians how to help patients manage pain, or enable access to alternative therapies.

So what happens? Addicted patients seeking to self-medicate their pain are turning to street drugs like heroin or synthetic fentanyl. In many cases these street drugs are far more powerful than users expect, and they can be lethal. As the NIH reported in May 2018, an analysis of opioid-related overdose deaths found that synthetic opioids including illicit fentanyl have surpassed prescription opioids as the most common drug involved in overdose deaths in the United States. Cutting off opioids used by addicted people hasn't made them healthier—it's merely forced them to ingest more dangerous street supplies like heroin and fentanyl, further increasing the death rate.

Doug: What is the difference between using low-level laser therapy and taking prescriptions of opioids or non-steroidal anti-inflammatory drugs to relieve pain?

Jim: Well, both of them relieve pain. So, people can look at both of them. But of course, I prefer low-level laser over drugs.

Doug: Is low-level laser safer than taking prescriptions opioids and NSAIDs?

Jim: Zero people die from low-level laser and there are no side effects. About 47,000 people die each year from taking pain killing drugs. So, a laser is a lot safer way to go.

Doug: What impact does laser and prescription of opioids and NSAIDs have on the digestive system?

Jim: Opioids wreak havoc on the digestive system. There are billions of nerves throughout the digestive system. Opioids block pain signals in your brain and other parts of the central nervous system by attaching to mu-receptors. But opioids don't discriminate, and they also attach to mu-receptors in the bowel. When you take opiates, they deaden the nerves and muscles of your digestive system, which is why opiate abusers often have severe constipation. Opioids are able to partially paralyze the stomach (gastroparesis) so that food remains in the digestive organ for a longer period of time. Opioids also reduce digestive secretions and decrease the urge to defecate. In fact, there's a new term for it: opioid-induced constipation (OIC). As many as 80% of people who take opioids for chronic, non-cancer pain experience constipation.

And guess what? That means you have to take another drug for your OIC! You've seen the ads on television and online for drugs like Movantik, which is specifically designed for OIC, and is supposed help you go more often by blocking opioids from binding to these mu-receptors in your bowel. So now you're taking more prescriptions!

This is the cascade effect, where you take a second drug to counteract the bad side effects of the first one. It's related to *polypharmacy,* a term used to describe the use of numerous medications at the same time (from the root "multiple pharmacies"). As people get older, they tend to have more health conditions that must be treated. Diagnosed with a range of issues from short-term medical conditions to chronic conditions like diabetes or high blood pressure, the senior citizen may be prescribed a wide variety of drugs at one time. Think about this: A study in 2010 found that the average 81-year-old was taking an average of 15 different medications at the same time, ranging from 6 to 28 medications. It's incredible how we've come to depend on pharmaceuticals, a trend that makes drug-free treatments including low-level laser all the more important. If low-level laser treatments can keep someone off prescription drugs, or on fewer prescription drugs, then isn't that worthwhile?

In contrast, the low-level laser is healing. It doesn't mess with your mu-receptors. So, if you're lasering, let's say, somebody's GI tract, you can be healing it. With the drugs, there can be constipation, nausea, vomiting, and other digestive disorders. Some people projectile vomit blood from taking NSAIDS. So laser is better for the GI tract versus drugs.

Doug: What's the difference in healing, comparing laser and prescription opioids and NSAIDs?

Jim: Well, laser heals all tissue: muscles, tendons, ligaments, bones, and brain tissue. It regenerates tissues. Drugs damage the GI tract, they don't heal. Laser helps the body with no side effects. Painkilling drugs are toxic, risky and dangerous. If people can look at the alternative to taking drugs, that will be quite good. If you are taking prescription opioids or non-steroidal anti-inflammatory drugs, please consider other healthy options, because drugs aren't good for your health.

Doug: A question came up about talking to my doctor about laser treatment. Is there something you should say to them? Or how do I present that to my physician?

Jim: Yes. That's a great idea. You can talk to your doctor about low-level laser therapy. Some medical doctors are using it. Harvard School of Medicine is using it. But most medical doctors aren't familiar with low-level laser therapy even though it's been around for fifty years. But for sure, you can ask them about it. Absolutely.

Chapter 3: Healthy Foods and Supplements

Doug: What are some other ways to get healthy pain relief and healing?

Jim: There's healthy food, there are nutritional supplements, and there are relaxing exercises that I can help people with.

Doug: What foods can I eat to help relieve pain?

Jim: Cherries are a very healthy, good thing to eat. Cherries can help with arthritis and muscle pain. Ginger can help with migraines, arthritis and sore muscles. Unsweetened cranberry juice can help with ulcers. Salmon is a superfood. It is great for your brain and your skin. It helps an achy back, neck, joints, and arthritis. Sardines also help with an achy back, neck, and joints. Turmeric is classic for pain relief. It assists with achy joints, arthritis, and colitis. Mint helps with irritable bowel syndrome and headaches. Edamame helps with arthritis. Hot chili peppers have capsaicin that helps with arthritis. These are some ideas I read in *Prevention* magazine.

Blueberries reduce inflammation. Pumpkin seeds are good for migraines. Virgin olive oil is good for the brain and joints. I glass of red wine is healthy and can help to ease disk swelling. Some of these ideas come from WebMD. Pineapple can help with arthritis. Apples can reduce inflammation. Brown rice can help with irritable bowel syndrome.

Doug: What foods should pain suffers avoid?

Jim: Avoid sugar, including fresh fruit juices. The increased insulin can worsen pain. Sugar is in many foods. Skip wheat. Wheat is bad for your GI tract, bad for your joints, and bad for your brain. You can notice a difference right away from stopping wheat and gluten. This is big. And you can lose weight by eliminating wheat from your diet. Wheat is in many man-made foods.

Avoid food with residual pesticides and chemicals. Avoid caffeine. This can disturb sleep. If you have to have caffeine, have one cup in the morning. Avoid nightshade vegetables. Tomatoes, potatoes, and eggplant may trigger arthritis. Avoid fried foods. These promote inflammation. Skip the French fries. Avoid aspartame. This artificial sweetener can increase your sensitivity to pain. Avoid monosodium glutamate (MSG). This can stimulate pain receptors. MSG is in many man-made foods. Some of these ideas are from Dr. Mercola.

The other thing to do is drink ½ your body weight in water each day. So I'm 150 pounds, which would be 75 ounces of water per day for me. This will help your body function and heal better.

Doug: Why should I change my diet?

Jim: When you eat more healthy foods and reduce the unhealthy foods, you will feel better. You will have less pain. You will heal faster. When you eliminate wheat, aspartame, and MSG, you can expect to feel better right away. You will have less fatigue and more energy. Wheat and sugar are many things. So check your labels and tell the servers at restaurants that you don't want sugar or wheat.

Apple cider vinegar can manage pain and reduce inflammation. Coconut oil can boost your immune system and reduce pain. Grapes and reduce inflammation, pain and swelling.

Doug: What's a good restaurant to go to in the Tucson area?

Jim: Govinda's Natural Foods Buffet in Tucson is wonderful. It is very healthy and vegetarian. It is the most peaceful and spiritual restaurant in Tucson also. The food is delicious. Vegetables, fruits, rice, beans, lentils and much more are on the buffet. Just remember to skip the items with wheat and sugar. They have a pond, turtles, love birds, and an excellent patio. The food is blessed. This place is great for healing and peacefulness.

Doug: Where is a healthy place to get groceries?

Jim: I love Whole Foods. You can eat there. They have a salad bar, hot bar, and deli. The ingredients of each item are listed. You can check for sugar and wheat. You can get gluten-free pizzas and sandwiches. You can get tacos. They also have soups without MSG. I like the chunky beef chili and the chicken tortilla soup.

The grocery store is terrific. There are lots of organic choices. You can find kale, collard greens, and arugula. You can find your organic blueberries here. They have sweet potatoes. You can find Nature's Way raw coconut. This is great for your brain. You can get your virgin olive oil. They have frozen fruits and vegetables too. These are great because there is no waste. You use what you want and refreeze the rest.

Doug: What is a good breakfast?

Jim: I like to do a vegetable and fruit smoothie. Add in some nutritional powders. Cherries or cherry juice, ginger, cranberries, turmeric, mint, edamame, and blueberries would be terrific. I would also add kale, spinach, collard greens, chard or arugula for a vegetable. I use Optimal Health Systems Complete Nutrition Plus too. One scoop is good. And Optimal Health Systems Fruit and Veggie Plus is wonderful. I use a scoop every day. This is the healthiest thing I eat every day.

I also eat eggs and gluten-free bread for breakfast.

Inflammation and Joint Pain

Doug: What nutritional supplements can I take to relieve pain and inflammation and heal?

Jim: Optimal Health Systems Joint Pak is a supplement we have been using and getting some good results. It reduces pain, inflammation, repairs tissue and repairs discs.

Here is what the company says about this supplement. You can read it at optimalhealthsysems.com:

> The Optimal Joint Pak combines the unique formulations of the Optimal Chronic and Optimal Acute in a convenient one-a-day packet. Optimal Chronic was created based on amazing research which proves

beyond question that specific nutrients will help repair disks and damaged tissue. Optimal Acute contains the proteolytic enzymes, minerals, herbs and antioxidants shown to have the most profound effect on the acute inflammatory response. Together these formulations help to aid the body in reducing tissue inflammation and repair tissue or disk degeneration.

Recommended Use: Take one packet daily between meals.

Do you know the number one reason Americans access the Healthcare System today? Pain, but not just any pain. Joint pain.

Every day millions of Americans struggle with inflammation leading to chronic aches and pains, and sore joints. The closest approximation is about 100 million Americans. That's more sufferers than diabetes, heart disease, and cancer combined. Combined! Even the simplest of daily tasks become a chore, not to mention physical activity being excruciatingly impossible.

Inflammation also has another effect as well. Any idea what it is? It just makes you feel like you're getting old. How many times have you clutched an ailing joint and said something like, "Ugh, I'm getting old." Who needs that? Are you someone who struggles with this daily? If so, you're just part of a growing number of Americans who have the same problem.

All that pain tallies up anywhere from $261 billion to $300 billion annually in health care bills. This translates into poorer performance at work, thus lower productivity, and lost wages. Pain is more than a debilitating problem. It has a quantifiable fiscal cost that affects all of us.

So, what can you do about it? If people turn to potentially harmful non-steroidal anti-inflammatory drugs (NSAIDs), they often do more harm than good. If you recall our discussion of NSAIDS, then you learned they block the natural healing process. This risk-versus-benefit factor of NSAIDS wasn't good enough for us at OHS. Still, we couldn't just let people suffer needlessly. There had to be a better answer found in nature.

The great news is we found it. There is another solution, a safe and natural one at that. In fact, there are a few solutions that can be combined in a few ways to meet your exact health needs. While pain is the same, everyone's bodies are different, and everyone needs their own TLC.

Your safe solution is the Optimal Joint Pak. It combines two of our pain and inflammation-relieving/healing products, Optimal Acute™ and Optimal Chronic™ into one affordable, portable Pak. With consultation from your health professional, a combination of both supplements are customized into dosages that fit your needs so you can move around with ease and enjoy life to the fullest again.

You can keep them handy if you go on a hike, work extra hard on manual labor, power through a tough workout, and so on. Together, these formulas help reduce inflammation and repair tissue and disc degeneration. You can use them on a daily basis, along with an extra packet when the need arises. The ingredients have been proven to be safer than NSAIDs and synthetic anti-inflammatories.

Jim: Optimal Health Systems Fruit and Veggie Plus is terrific also. I take it every day. Optimal Fruit & Veggie Plus is a highly potent antioxidant powder with 24 raw freeze dried fruits and vegetables. These are combined with organic juices, herbs, and natural flavorings to provide a great-tasting powder. One serving of Optimal Fruit & Veggie Plus has over 13 times the antioxidant potency than the average American gets per day. That is 20,000 antioxidant ORAC units per serving.

It helps with cancer, degenerative diseases, and overall body inflammation. It promotes cardiovascular health, healthy glucose metabolism, healthy vision, healthy inflammatory response and healthy brain function. It also provides healthy aging. It supports healthy immune response, healthy skin, and a healthy urinary tract.

Relaxing Exercises

Doug: Are there relaxing exercises that can help me feel more comfortable?

Jim: I've been using Feldenkrais exercises for 30 years to relieve pain, increase the range of motion and to be more comfortable. I have used them for myself, my family and with other people.

The Feldenkrais method is the invention of Israeli physicist Moshe Feldenkrais. He developed a way of "retraining" the body. There are two modes of this retraining.

The first is group classes called Awareness Through Movement or ATMs, which resemble yoga or tai chi classes, but are very different. For example, the instructor makes no movements; rather, he or she talks while *you* do the movements. The second mode involves one-on-one sessions, called functional integration, or FI, with a trained practitioner. In such a session you lie fully clothed on a low table and the practitioner gently moves or presses your body in different directions to make you aware of the subconscious tension and holding patterns that make your movement less efficient, as well as more efficient ways of coordinating your body.

They are easy. You'll learn to use your body in a new way. You do less than stretching, and it's gentle. A feature of the Feldenkrais method is the emphasis on doing movements extremely slowly and gently, which is essential for releasing yourself from habitual movement patterns and then learning new ones. The focus on slow movement also makes it ideal for older people or those who are in chronic pain. To benefit from the method, you don't have to have an understanding of a complex system. All that is required is to do slow, careful movement, while paying close attention to things pointed out by your teacher. Another healthy feature of the method is that it discourages mindless repetition or any kind of macho attitude. It's all about exploring, and it's fine if no two movements are the same.

I use the exercises to help heal people. I am not a licensed Feldenkrais practitioner. I searched for licensed Feldenkrais practitioners in Tucson at Feldenkrais.com and did not find anyone. I can help you relax and increase your range of motion.

Your Visit to the Doctor Begins With Conversation

Doug: When I go to the doctor, I spend so little time face-to-face with a physician. They hardly seem to have a minute to talk about stuff. They don't even have time to answer my questions. So, I'm interested in how the laser can help me before I see the doctor next time.

Jim: That's good. Thank you for that question, Doug. That's right. In 2007, researcher Ming Tai-Seale and others decided to find out the duration of the average doctor visit. In their paper "Time Allocation in Primary Care Office Visits," they reviewed nearly 400 videotaped office visits. In their words, they found a "very limited amount of time was dedicated to specific topics in office visits." The median duration of an office visit was only 15.7 minutes, covering a median of six topics. Only about five minutes were spent on the longest topic, and the remaining topics each received a median of only 1.1 minutes. They noted that the length of the visit overall varied little even when contents of visits varied widely. The researchers concluded, "Efforts to improve the quality of care need to recognize the time pressure on both patients and physicians, the effects of financial incentives, and the time costs of improving patient–physician interactions."

Most medical doctors are busy, so they've got a short amount of time to spend with you. I enjoy being with people, so I've got more time to spend with them. I like talking about the issues people have. I'll ask, "What kind of pain do you have?" We treat them in those areas they're in pain or have soreness. We also talk about diet all the time, like "are you drinking your water?" We talk about exercise. They say they've got this issue, and so we have a conversation. I love spending time with people.

People bring different issues they have with their health. For some people, like the woman with the tendinitis, two treatments and she was done. For other people, maybe they need to do a couple of times a month. It depends on the situation and how many issues people have. If you have one issue or a small pain, the time for healing won't be as much as someone who has eight different issues. Some people have problems with their shoulders, their neck, their knees, their ankles and their feet. I have clients like that, you know, and that can be an ongoing opportunity.

Doug: Why should I come to you versus seeing a medical doctor, seeing someone else, or doing nothing?

Jim: In some cases, a medical doctor is the way to go. But traditional practitioners tend to have fallback positions. They're short on time, so they gravitate towards the most expedient solution. Often this involves writing a prescription.

I won't drug you as the first option. I can probably relieve your pain and inflammation. You will probably have pain relief at your first treatment. You will receive healing. Your treatment will be relaxing, calming and comfortable. The first treatment is free. I guarantee my work. You either benefit or it is free. I can come to your home or you can come to two office locations I have. Your treatment is non-toxic with no side effects. I can treat at least four locations on your body that are uncomfortable. Your range of motion will be improved. You will have increased blood circulation. We can probably get you back to doing the things you like to do, like walking, exercising, dancing and golfing. We can probably keep you active.

Doug: Thanks for helping me heal from injuries.

Jim: It has been a pleasure to help you to heal. You're 69 nine years old, you exercise, you do Pilates twice a week, you do yoga, and you do a dance class. You're a big guy. You're able to stay active. The laser has relieved your pain healed you. That's awesome that you are so active.

Doug: Oh, and my back is sore.

Jim: It's funny because it's Thursday and you just had all your exercise classes this week. Now your back is sore!

Eat Healthy, Get Exercise

Doug: What can I do to relieve my back pain or knee pain?

Jim: First, eat a healthy diet for your body. Cherries, ginger, salmon, sardines, turmeric, edamame, hot chili peppers, virgin olive oil, and red wine can all help. Avoid sugar. Avoid wheat like the plague. Skip tomatoes, potatoes, and eggplant. Skip French fries and other fried food. Avoid aspartame and MSG. Come see me. We'll laser you and do some relaxing exercises to relieve pain and help you heal. You will also receive Optimal Health Systems Joint Pak for healthy pain relief and healing.

Doug: So how can people in pain get comfortable again? How can they be active, exercise, walk, dance and golf again?

Jim: Ok. Eat healthy foods daily, drink your water daily, exercise daily, and go for walks.

Walking is a great exercise. Regular walking can help improve your body's response to insulin, which can help reduce belly fat. Walking every day is one of the most effective low-impact ways to positively alter body composition and mobilize fat. Daily walking increases metabolism by burning extra calories and by preventing muscle loss, which is particularly important as you get older. And to see these benefits, you don't have to drive to the gym. I knew a person who in just one month reduced her body fat by four percent. She did this by walking home from work each day, which was just under a mile. That was all. She didn't do anything else except walk ten minutes to work and ten minutes home.

It gets better. The American Diabetes Association says walking lowers your blood sugar levels and your overall risk for diabetes. Researchers have found that regular walking lowers blood pressure by as much as 11 points and may reduce the risk of stroke by as much as forty percent. Walking helps your appearance too—it drains the lower legs of excess fluid and can help prevent varicose veins through the pumping action of the calf muscles. Plus, exercise promotes the increased supply of oxygen, which also gets rid of the waste products in the tissues.

Every day, take some good, targeted nutritional supplements. Do some relaxing exercises daily. And get low-level laser treatments as necessary for pain relief and healing. You're going to be healthier, more active and feel better. You'll have more energy and you can get back to do what you want to do in your life.

Chapter 4: Breathing Exercises

Breathing exercises can help you relax and heal. You can use them to reduce suffering. You can reduce the tension in your body. You can find and discover your inner peace. You can energize yourself. And you can reduce your pain. You will get more oxygen into your body. Your immune system will be boosted. Breathing exercises improve your physical and emotional health. They can be meditations.

One of the keys is to exhale more than you inhale. Exhale out the stale air in your lungs. You will naturally breathe in fresh new oxygen. Inhale through the nose and exhale through the mouth.

Breathing exercises activate the parasympathetic nervous system. This helps you relax and heal. You want to activate the relaxing glands of your body.

One of the keys is to keep breathing. Don't hold your breath. And don't take shallow breaths. Keep breathing and keep getting oxygen into your body. Exhale as much as you can.

Laughter is a fun way to exhale, to get more oxygen and get more energy. So laugh for as long as you can.

Here are three breathing exercises from yoga. These can help you relax and feel better.

The first one is humming. This is simple. You just hum. Please try it. Take a long deep breath in through your nose. While exhaling, hum it out by closing your lips slightly. While you are humming, feel the vibrations in your facial muscles, your skull and deep into your brain cells. Be aware of your head. You can do this in two ways. One is without blocking the ears and one is with blocking the ear canals. You can block your ears with your fingers. When you block your ears, you can hear the deep humming into your brain cells. Please close your eyes, take a long, deep breath, and hum it out. Keep humming as long as possible until you run out of breath. You want to get the stale air out of your lungs. Take your time to fill up your lungs and do it again. No rush, don't be in a hurry. Relax. Keep on changing the pitch and tone of your humming. Go high and low, and see with which frequency, pitch, and tone you feel the most relaxed. Do low humming, high pitch. Try a low pitch. Keep experimenting and find what has the most relaxation for you. This has a lulling effect on the brain cells. It is good for insomnia and memory. Humming is a very powerful relaxing exercise. It brings down your breathing rate, heart rate, and blood pressure. You can do it for 5 to 30 minutes.

Another powerful breathing exercise is "synchronized breathing," or "belly breathing." Normally we adults breathe from our chest. But when children breathe, their abdomen is moving up and down all the time. Children don't breathe from their chest. This is the healthy way to breathe. We are relearning here how to breathe from our abdomen. You want to move your diaphragm. The diaphragm is a sheet of internal skeletal muscle that extends across the bottom of the thoracic cavity. The diaphragm separates the thoracic cavity, containing the heart and lungs, from the abdominal cavity. It performs an important function in respiration: as the diaphragm contracts, the volume of the thoracic cavity increases and air is drawn into the lungs.

When you inhale, put your hand on your belly. Act as if there is a balloon inside your abdomen and inflate the balloon. When you exhale, the abdomen goes down. Inhale through your nose and exhale through your mouth. When you inhale, your abdomen comes up. Please try it. When you exhale from your mouth, you can exhale longer. Always inhale from the nose. Exhale like you are blowing air. Please close your eyes and do it ten times.

Synchronized breathing is a very powerful exercise to use when your mind is in turmoil. You can breathe from your abdomen 20 times and become peaceful. Breathing from the diaphragm activates the vagus nerve, which stimulates the parasympathetic system. This brings down the heart rate and breathing rate. It brings down the blood pressure and reduces the stress level. It is a quick way to calm down when you are angry or upset.

The last breathing exercise is "mindful breathing," or "total body breathing." Normally we breathe from the lungs. Here, we imagine that we are breathing from the entire body. The air you inhale goes to your head, arms, chest, waist, feet, and everywhere. Your whole body expands when you breathe in, and your whole body deflates like a balloon when you exhale. Sit with your spine and back erect. Please try it. Close your eyes. When you are breathing in, imagine that you are breathing from each and every part of your body. The entire body is breathing. When you inhale, your body is expanding like a balloon. When you exhale, your body is relaxing and deflating. When you exhale, relax all of the muscles of your body. Breathe into any part of your body where there is discomfort. Heal this part of your body. Relax that area. I find this very relaxing. This ties in well with the inner body meditation.

When you do these three breathing exercises, you will have more energy. You will feel relaxed. Your pain can be reduced. You can eliminate your suffering.

I learned these three breathing exercises from Dr. Madan Kataria, the founder and originator of the worldwide Laughter Yoga Movement. There's much more about the healing power of laughter in the pages ahead.

Chapter 5: Mimi's Low-Level Laser Success Story

Mimi came to me on November 28, 2017. Her issues included depression, lumbar stenosis, rotator cuff damage, sinusitis, ankle pain and hip pain. She had surgery done on her low back in October 2016. She also had an ankle replacement in March 2017.

We treated her that day for her lower back, hip, and ankle. After the laser treatment, her lower back was better on the right side; and, was same on the left side, her hips were better and her ankle was a lot better. The ankle was not as swollen.

December 5. I lasered her mid back, lower back, ankle, hips and left ankle. The lower back and ankle had less pain afterwards. We did some Feldenkrais exercises and inner body meditation.

December 12. She was distraught and depressed. She had injured her back bowling. I lasered her back, hips, ankle and foot.

December 15. She had neck low back, hips, and ankle and foot issues. I lasered her issues.   Everything was better, especially her hips.

January 12, 2018. She started taking Optimal Health Systems Joint Pak and Fruit and Veggie Plus. She had some anxiety. I lasered her forehead, neck, shoulders, mid back, low back, and foot.

January 16. She appeared to be depressed. I lasered her forehead, neck, shoulders, low back, foot, and heart. She had some sinusitis. Her pain was lowered after the treatment and she felt at peace.

January 26. She started taking Optimal Health Systems Flora (probiotics). She also did an infrared sauna. I lasered her neck, low back, ankle, and foot.

March 6. I lasered her forehead, back of head, neck, sinuses, right shoulder (rotator cuff), ankle and foot. She did a sauna.

April 3. I lasered her forehead, back of head, sinuses, shoulders, low back, and hips. The left shoulder and left hip were better. We did some breathing exercises. She did a sauna. The next day, the left shoulder and back were much better. The right shoulder and hip were somewhat better.

April 10. I lasered the forehead, back of head, sinuses, neck, both shoulders, low back, hips, and feet. We did some Feldenkrais and breathing exercises. She did a sauna. Everything was better!

April 17. I lasered her forehead, back of head, sinuses, neck, shoulders, low back, hips, ankles, and feet. We did some Feldenkrais and she did a sauna. Everything was better.

April 25. I lasered her forehead, back of head, sinuses, right shoulder, low back, hips, left ankle, feet, and toes. She did a sauna. We did some Feldenkrais and she did a Bemer treatment at the same time.

She has been swimming again.

On May 15, 2018, she gave me her testimonial:

October, 2016, I had back surgery for stenosis; and, March, 2017, I had a total left ankle replacement, which was a major operation. After both operations I had some pain in my neck, lower back, and left ankle. I've had nine treatments from Jim, and my swelling, redness, and discomfort have become eliminated in my left ankle, neck and back since my treatments. I had total success with my ankle, neck and back issues. With his treatments I have become more positive and happier. I recommend Jim for any pain you may have. He has even helped my sinus issues!!!! Thank you! MiMi Battin

She told me today she has no pain in her body!

Chapter 6: A Healthy and Healing Day

Here's a schedule for a healthy and healing day! Of course, this is just a suggestion, and you can personalize it to fit your lifestyle.

Morning

Drink 36+ ounces of water in the morning.

Go for a walk in the sun.

Eat a breakfast that includes:

Fruit and vegetable drink: organic cherries or organic cherry juice, ginger, unsweetened cranberry juice, turmeric, mint. Add your favorite vegetable.

Take your Optimal Health Systems Joint Pak supplements.

Midday

Make a contribution to others in a way that is satisfying for you.

Laugh often throughout the day.

Eat a healthy lunch that includes: salmon, edamame, and a salad with olive oil.

Do a breathing exercise.

Drink 36+ ounces of water in the afternoon.

Evening

Meditate.

Eat dinner that includes hot chili peppers, such as Mexican food, and enjoy one glass of red wine.

Drink 8 ounces of water.

Do some relaxing exercises on your back to heal your body.

Example of an Unhealthy, Pain-Creating Day

Just as you can create a healthy day of joy and the celebration of life, it's also within your power to create a day that's full of pain and suffering. You wouldn't think you'd ever want to do this… but how many times have you found yourself doing things that create pain?

Drink no water.

Have a breakfast that includes wheat cereal with sugar.

Go to a job you don't like.

Eat a lunch that includes a hamburger, French fries, and Diet Coke with aspartame.

Sit at a desk for four hours, staring at a computer screen.

Eat a dinner that includes Chinese food with MSG.

Watch a movie with gratuitous and pointless violence or scenes of hatred.

Go to bed angry.

Forget to do your breathing exercises or meditate on the blessings of life.

Forget to express gratitude.

Chapter 7: The Benefits of Laughter

Laughter is another way to relieve emotional and physical pain. Laughter can release happy hormones and chemicals in your body. The idea is to laugh as often as you can for as long as you can. Any time you get a chance to laugh, take it. I laugh when other people are laughing. I laugh even if I don't know what they are laughing about. Laughter is stress relieving. It brings you into the present moment. You can experience peace and joy. The more you laugh, the happier you will be. I laugh in the shower every day. That comes with practice. And I lead laughter sessions.

One easy way to laugh is to laugh anytime someone tells a joke. Laugh even if the joke is not funny. You will feel better. You can laugh at the absurdities of life. Everything is laughable. We take things way to serious. I laugh at myself when I trip on the sidewalk. It is OK to be human. Laughing is healing. It is a victory. Laughter breaks anxiety.

"It only hurts when I am not laughing," said film actor Jackie Chan. How true!

You can certainly watch a funny half-hour show on television to get some laughs. You can watch comedians on YouTube. It is great to have a friend who makes you laugh.

Laughter strengthens the immune system. It helps your creativity. It helps lighten your life. It can relieve your pain. You can relieve tension and stress. It also helps you keep perspective. You can enjoy your life more. Victor Borge said, "Laughter is the shortest distance between two people." It brings you closer to people. It brings you into the present moment. It boosts your life satisfaction. It helps you relax.

Here's a line from Groucho Marx that will make you laugh: "From the moment I picked your book up until I laid it down, I was convulsed with laughter. Someday, I intend to read it."

Kids laugh on the playground. They don't need jokes, humor or comedy. They just laugh. You can too. Laughter is ultimately a choice. The best laughter is to laugh at our problems. That releases stress. You can't laugh without being present.

"To truly laugh, you must be able to take your pain and play with it," said Charlie Chaplin.

You don't need a reason to laugh. You can laugh anytime you want. You can laugh because you want to feel more comfortable.

"If I get big laughs, I'm a comedian. If I get little laughs, I'm a humorist. If I get no laughs, I'm a singer," said George Burns

Thanks to Dr. Annette Goodheart for some of these ideas! She wrote the best selling book, *Laughter Therapy: How to Laugh About Everything in Your Life That Isn't Really Funny.* She's a pioneer in helping people throughout the world embrace the healing power of laughter. She has developed techniques that have allowed her clients to heal deep emotional wounds before moving on to happier and healthier living. In her book she explains that her goal is to empower her readers to bring more healing laughter into their lives and to become "laughter independent."

She outlines three myths about laughter that keep us from laughing.

The first myth is that we must have a reason to laugh. You don't need any reason at all, other than the joy of being alive!

The second myth is that we laugh because we are happy. We can laugh anytime!

The third myth is that a sense of humor is the same thing as laughter. She dispels these myths and reveals what she believes to be the reality of laughter—it's a powerful tonic for the soul.

And thanks also to Dr. Madan Kataria, the founder and originator of the worldwide Laughter Yoga Movement. Started with just five people in a public park in Mumbai in 1995, it has grown into a worldwide movement of more than 6,000 Laughter Yoga clubs in over 60 countries.

He teaches there's a big difference between *happiness* and *joy*.

Happiness is a conditional, temporary response subject to the fulfillment of our desires. We are happy when we get what we want, which means that our happiness depends upon external conditions. It's a conditional response—that is, if a certain condition is fulfilled, then we will be happy. But even if the anticipated conditions are fulfilled, happiness is often fleeting as it is quickly displaced by a new expectation of some event that will bring us happiness.

Happiness that lasts is never found because it's impossible to get happy and stay happy. If life is based on obtaining happiness, then we will always fall short because life is always changing.

In contrast, joy is internal and eternal. It's your unconditional commitment to have fun from within, regardless of outside conditions. It is an emotion that can be created by indulging in joyful activities like singing, dancing, playing, and laughing.

Dr. Kataria teaches that Laughter Yoga separates you from your memories and expectations. It makes it easier to handle the many challenges of life because it puts you strongly "in the moment," and it's when you're in the moment that you're not thinking about your problems. It's as if you literally cast them aside. Laughter lightens up your life and gives you an inner coping strength.

Laughter Yoga has measurable health benefits. It helps decrease stress, improve the immune system, increase circulation of blood flow, and improve overall health. It reduces the levels of stress-related hormones and neuropeptides and replaces these with happiness-related hormones and neuropeptides. By stressing deep diaphragmatic breathing, laughing fully oxygenates the bloodstream and major organs, thus providing a complete sense of well being.

Take a moment right now to put down this book and start laughing! It doesn't matter whether you have anything to laugh about. Just do it! If you need to close the door to avoid puzzled looks from your family or co-workers, go ahead. You can tell them you read something funny in a book, or you saw a funny kitten video on YouTube. Or better yet, just tell them you were laughing because you felt like it!

Chapter 8: Meditation

Meditation can be a way to access to peace, relaxation, and pain relief. Your whole life can be a meditation. This can bring you into the present moment. You can feel calm and serene. When you are at peace, your body can heal. If you are anxious, it is harder for your body to repair itself.

There are dozens of ways to meditate. Some are ancient and some are modern, but any of them will work for you if you approach it with sincerity and conviction.

One thing that has greatly helped me is the spiritual acceptance that we—all of us—are eventually going to die. Accepting this fact can be very liberating. There is a death meditation, where you meditate on your own death. In Buddhism, the practice of death meditation is common. It's called Maranasati, and in the words of the Buddha, "of all the footprints, that of the elephant is supreme. Similarly, of all mindfulness meditation, that on death is supreme."

Eckhart Tolle likes to go to cemeteries. I took my nine-year-old son to a cemetery when we were on a vacation. He is glad we went. It shows you the impermanence of everything, and us.

Scientists usually classify meditation based on the way they focus attention, into two categories: focused attention and open monitoring.

Focused attention meditation means keeping your thoughts on a single object during the meditation session. This object may be the breath, a mantra, visualization, part of the body, or external object. Examples of this include Samatha (Buddhist meditation), chakra meditation, Kundalini meditation, mantra meditation, Pranayama, and many others.

A mantra is a syllable or word, usually without any particular meaning, that is repeated for the purpose of focusing your mind. It's not supposed to change you or convince you of something. For example, "I will be a better person" is not a mantra in the meditative sense because it's presented in the *future tense*, which creates tension, contradicting the purpose of meditation. But a personal mantra can be a positive phrase or affirmative statement that you say to yourself for the purpose of motivation or encouragement. This could be your favorite quote, proverb, spiritual truth, or religious saying that motivates and inspires you to be your best self. It could be something like, "I have the light of the sun within me," because it's centered *on the present*. You're saying, "This is who I am *right now*."

Some practitioners say that the choice of word and its correct pronunciation are very important, due to the "vibration" associated to the sound and meaning. Others say that the mantra itself is only a tool to focus the mind, and the chosen word is irrelevant. You should do what's most comfortable for you.

As Deepak Chopra wrote, "As you repeat the mantra, it creates a mental vibration that allows the mind to experience deeper levels of awareness. As you meditate, the mantra becomes increasingly abstract and indistinct, until you're finally led into the field of pure consciousness from which the vibration arose."

Some of the most well known mantras from the Hindu and Buddhist traditions include:

- om

- so-ham

- om namah shivaya

- om mani padme hum

- rama

- yam

- ham

Open monitoring meditation means being aware all aspects of our experience, without attachment or judgment. All perceptions, be they external (sounds, smells) or internal (feelings, thoughts, memories) are recognized and accepted for what they are. They are what they are, and will enter and leave the mind on their own accord. Examples include mindfulness meditation, Vipassana, and some types of Taoist meditation.

Mindfulness meditation is the practice of intentionally focusing on the present moment, accepting and non-judgmentally paying attention to the sensations, thoughts, and emotions that arise. You can practice mindfulness during your daily activities: while eating, walking, and talking. For daily life meditation, the practice is to pay attention to what is going on in the present moment, to be aware of what is happening all around you, and not cruising on autopilot.

In-Out Meditation

A simple meditation to do is the **in-out meditation**.

Follow your breathing. As you breathe out, notice that it is your outgoing breath. As you breathe in, notice that it is your incoming breath. Please do it now. You are just following your breathing. You are putting your attention in your body. You take attention out of your mind. You are coming into the present moment, where your life is. So follow your breath. Feel the air as it moves through your nose and throat. You can take a moment and practice this. It will probably be easier to close your eyes as you do this. Notice what is happening to your shoulders. Are they moving? Can you feel anything in your belly? Just follow your breath. I find it very relaxing right now as I am doing it too. You will get better with practice. Clear your thoughts. When a thought comes up, just let it go and go back to your breathing. Be aware of your breathing. Notice your respiration.

This meditation can help you come out of the past. You can stop living in the future. You can connect with your life in the here and now. You can find peace in the present moment. You can relax and heal. As you breathe in, notice that you are breathing in. As you breathe out, notice that you are breathing out. Put your awareness in your body. Get out of your mind and thoughts. Connect with life. Feel the air filling your lungs. However, you are breathing is fine. No matter what is going on with us in our thoughts and emotions, our breathing is always with us like a faithful friend. When you feel anxious or stressed, you can return to your breathing. Notice the flow of air coming in and going out of your nose. You can do this conscious breathing anytime. You can do it while driving, while lying in bed, while walking, anytime. I use it throughout the day.

We think too much. Be aware of what is happening with your breath. Reunite your mind and body. It's very important to go home to the present moment to get in touch with the healing, refreshing and nourishing elements of life inside and around you. You can be free from your resentments, worries, and fears. You get in touch with your body. Your body is a wonder. When you follow your breath, you come into the here and now. You get in touch with life.

In the beginning, you may notice that your breathing may feel labored or awkward. Your breath is a result of your body and feelings. If your body has tension or pain, then your breath is affected. Don't force your breath. However, you are breathing is fine. Let it be. Just become aware of your breath. After some time, the quality of your breathing will improve naturally. After one or two minutes, notice that the quality of your breathing improves. Your in-breath will become deeper. Your out-breath will become slower. Your breathing becomes more peaceful and harmonious.

Frequently, we neglect and ignore our body. Now is a chance to come home to your body and make friends with it.

If you want, you can put your hand on your belly. You'll notice when you breathe in, your stomach is rising. When you breathe out, your belly is falling. Be aware of your in breath and out breath from beginning to end. Enjoy it. You don't have to think about your pain, your suffering, your past or your future. Breathing is pleasurable.

The present moment is the only moment that is real.

The more you practice this, the better you will get at it.

I learned in-out meditation from Thich Nhat Hanh, and have used many of his wonderful ideas here.

Inner Body Meditation

The **inner body meditation** is another way to find your inner peace, to relax and to relieve pain and suffering. Please take a few minutes to do this. You are taking your attention out of the mind and putting it into the body. Feel your body from within. Anything you notice is great. Maybe you can feel your hands. Maybe you can feel your right foot. Anything you feel is great. Put your attention into your body.

And attempt to feel your whole body. If you feel your hands, then notice your wrists too. Feel your wrists. Be aware of your hands and wrists. Feel your lower arm. Feel our biceps and triceps. Be aware of your arms. Take the attention out if your mind and thoughts and put it into your body. Feel your arms. Notice your shoulders. Feel them move as you breathe. Notice your neck. Do you feel any tension? Feel your jaw. Feel your face and scalp. Put your attention in your body. Notice your chest. Is it moving? Feel your belly. Can you sense movement in your belly? Feel your pelvis. Be aware of your back. Get out of your thoughts and be in your body. Inhabit the body. Be aware of your torso. Feel your thighs. Notice your calves. Feel your feet and toes. Be aware of your whole body. Let go of your thoughts. Come into the body. Feel your body breathing.

Now notice any energy in your body. Is your body alive? Is there pulsing? Feel the relaxation. Let go of your thoughts. Heal your body. Breathe into any area of your body that has pain. Feel the life force in your body. Where do you notice it? I can feel the inner smile. Be in touch with your body. Connect to the energy. Feel the life force. Notice if you can feel the energy in your whole body. Feel the relaxation. Notice any pulsation.

If all you feel is your right foot, great. If you can feel the life force in your whole body, that is great.

I do this meditation every day. It helps with keeping perspective. I feel connected to energy. Clients say it is very powerful for them.

You can feel a deep sense of peace and grounding. You get in touch with yourself and the life force.

I learned this meditation from Eckhart Tolle. It is the most powerful thing I do.

Chapter 9: Pain, Suffering, and Joy

"Pain is inevitable; suffering is optional." – ancient Buddhist proverb.

What is the difference between pain and suffering?

If you have physical pain, then that is the way it is. If you back pain is a five on a scale of 1-10, then that is what you are experiencing. That is what is.

If you are upset because your back hurts, then that is *suffering,* and is unnecessary. The opportunity is to separate the physical pain from the emotional suffering.

If you can accept what is, then you don't need to suffer. OK, there is physical pain. You can choose to accept that. Not that you are happy about it. Of course you are not happy about it. The suffering is unnecessary. So the challenge is to separate pain from suffering. Accept that you have pain at this moment.

Don't accept that you will have pain the rest of your life. No. Accept that you have it now, this second. You can choose to do something about it.

You can call me to help, for example. So that is the challenge for us each moment. To accept what is, at that moment.

"The difference between pain and suffering is the difference between what is and what you want it to be," said author Stephen Levine.

Being Joyful Despite Pain and Adversity

As a pain relief specialist, it's my job to deliver my clients from physical pain. I enjoy my work and I've helped many people. But along the way I've also noticed something: some people who are in pain nevertheless have a surprisingly positive outlook on life. Nothing dampens their spirits! And conversely, I've known many people who are in perfect health and free of pain and who, for some reason, are miserable. They suffer even though they have no pain.

That's why this book includes information and advice on how to live a life not of just happiness, which is fleeting, but of deep joy, which lasts forever.

I knew a woman who was in her nineties. Alice still lived in her own home and, with help from her daughter, took care of herself. And she loved life! If you saw her and asked her how she felt, she would reply, "Never better!" You would think she had lived a charmed life. In fact, Alice had experienced her fair share of pain. Her husband had died in a terrible car accident. Her house had once burned down—it was in the path of a forest fire, and nothing could be done to stop it—and she had lost everything. Her other daughter had died of cancer when only in her twenties. She herself was nearly blind and had crippling arthritis that made every movement difficult. But yet these sources of pain never seemed to matter. Alice saw her mission as helping others to be happy, and all the obstacles that life threw in her way could be pushed aside.

When you're in chronic pain, it can be very difficult to think positively, look on the bright side, and find your inner joy. Nobody will ever tell you that it's easy. However, there are people who suffer adversity and who yet consistently express feelings of contentment and inner joy. Like Alice, they're people who have made the conscious choice to be joyful in life.

What's the secret? Here are four traits that chronically ill people who are joyful have in common:

1. Acceptance – Among chronic illness patients, the ones who stay focused on the good things in their lives recover quicker than those who choose to dwell only on their misfortunes. Like my friend Alice, when you ask them about some terrible event in their lives, they'll shrug and say, "Things happen to everybody. You just have to do your best and keep moving." They don't ruminate over past injustices or injuries. They "go with the flow."

2. Hope – Chronically ill people who think that the future will be better are more likely to overcome their illnesses than those who are mired in the past, becoming depressed and despondent. Anxiety, depression, and stress conspire to make any pain you have feel more acute. Thinking positive thoughts about tomorrow not only makes you more joyous today, but it also helps to create a happier tomorrow.

3. Perseverance – Among people who are chronically ill yet joyful, another common trait is the determination to overcome adversity.

That's because to give in to the pain means sinking into regret and despair, which is a sure-fire recipe for a life of unhappiness. When "up" is the only way to go, the people who persevere make it to the top.

4. Empathy – When you care about others and identify with their pain, you worry less about your own. I see so many people who are fixated on their own problems, and it almost seems normal until I meet the Iraq War veteran who lost both his legs and who tells me he's going to help a buddy "who's much worse off" (he says) climb a mountain in the Rockies. Then I realize what problems really mean! It's hard to be unhappy while you're reaching out to help somebody else who is in need.

Chapter 10: Start Walking!

Walking can be a great way to relieve both pain and suffering. It can also help you feel more comfortable and relaxed. You can come into the present moment. You can get some Vitamin D from the sun. You connect with the peace of nature. I love to walk and do it most days of the week. You can find and discover your inner peace and joy. You can relieve tension. It is a great exercise. It is good for your joints and muscles. It helps digestion. It improves your circulation.

One reason why walking is necessary is that as a society we are becoming increasingly sedentary. From an evolutionary perspective, in the blink of an eye we've gone from living as: 1) physically active hunter-gatherers in the wild, to 2) physically active farmers and factory workers, and then to 3) office workers spending our days sitting in comfortable chairs inside large apartment complexes and office buildings. After spending eight hours sitting in office cubicles staring at computers, we get into our cars and drive home, where we eat dinner before sitting some more in front of the television set. "Physical inactivity is pandemic today," as the authoritative British medical journal *The Lancet* put it in a special issue devoted to the benefits of physical activity.

Another way of saying it is, "Sitting is the new smoking." Just as smoking cigarettes was seen as a totally pointless way to shorten your life, so is being sedentary. A good way to stay healthy is to *keep walking*.

As *The New York Times* reported in 2010, many health experts encourage people to walk 10,000 steps per day, which is about five miles. The Centers for Disease Control and Prevention puts it differently—they recommend adults engage in 150 minutes of moderate activity a week, such as brisk walking. To meet the CDC's recommendation, you need to walk about 7,000 to 8,000 steps a day. Researchers say it takes roughly 2,000 steps to reach a mile. But the average American only walks about half the recommended amount of 10,000 steps, according to Catrine Tudor-Locke, director of the Walking Behavior Laboratory at Pennington Biomedical Research Center. She told Live Science.com that the typical American takes about 5,900 steps a day.

The American champions of walking? A 2004 study in the journal *Medicine & Science in Sports & Exercise* found that male adults in Amish farming communities took more than 18,000 steps, while female Amish people averaged more than 14,000 daily. Compared with mainstream Americans, Plain Sect communities " have a significant edge in late-life health, with lower rates of cancer, cardiovascular disease, diabetes and more," *Time* magazine reported. The 2018 article by Jeffrey Kluger identified several lifestyle factors that likely play a role. The Amish are much more physically active than the average American, and their rates of obesity are far less. Including other forms of manual labor such as planting, chopping, lifting, and sowing, the Amish are six times as active as a random sample of people from 12 countries. Few Amish smoke, and their rates of smoking-related cancers are correspondingly low.

Studies published in leading medical journals show that walking and other physical activity could cut rates of diabetes, depression, breast and colon cancer, high blood pressure, cardiovascular disease, obesity, anxiety, and osteoporosis by at least 40 percent, according to the American College of Sports Medicine. This would save Americans more than $100 billion a year in health care costs, according to the American Public Health Association.

I encourage you to walk every day. Forty-five minutes or more is great. Five minutes is also good. My dad used to park one mile from the office and walk to work every day. My family would often walk to the end of the street after dinner. Anything is good.

No matter how much you walk, the most important thing is to increase your activity beyond what you were doing before. If you walked ten minutes yesterday, try to walk for fifteen minutes today.

There's hope that Americans may increase their walking due to advances in city planning. Fifty years ago, the automobile was king, and cities and suburbs were designed to accommodate motor vehicles while minimizing pedestrian traffic. No one was encouraged to walk! Now we realize that walking should be a natural part of our daily lives, rather than something we add on specifically for exercise, health, or recreation. If you live in a well-designed neighborhood, every day you can walk to the store, to the park, the dry cleaners, or the post office. The traditional common-sense idea of "walkability" is the result of deliberate urban planning that locates important destinations within walking distance, which is at the heart of making our communities more comfortable, safe, and convenient for walking.

While you are walking, it helps to come into the present moment. You can use your sense perceptions. Look at the sky, the plants, and animals. Listen for the wind or a bird. Feel the breeze and the temperature. Get out of your mind and thoughts.

Reconnecting with the natural world is important. In fact, there's a name for our current disconnect from nature: "Paleo-deficit disorder." Introduced by Alan C. Logan, Martin A. Katzman, and Vicent Balanzá-Martínez in their paper entitled, "Natural environments, ancestral diets, and microbial ecology: is there a modern 'paleo-deficit disorder'?" the idea is that our human-made environment has evolved much faster than we have, and as a result we're like a species living in an alien environment. The research focuses in particular on how changes in the human diet over the past several millennia have affected our health and how inadequate exposure to microorganisms can cause chronic low-grade inflammation and disease.

We strive to live in germ-free environments. The air we breathe in office buildings has been scrubbed clean of every spore and dust particle. After being inundated with advertisements urging us to kill every microbe and insect in our homes, we do this, with the result that we live in what anyone living a hundred years ago would think was an amazingly sterile environment. We compulsively use hand sanitizers. And worst of all, when we get a cold we run to the doctor and demand antibiotics to kill the nasty germs in our bodies.

Unfortunately, we also kill all the good germs that help us digest our food. We kill the germs that help strengthen our immune systems. In western societies, allergies have become epidemic. As *The New York Times* reported, depending on the study and population, the prevalence of allergic disease and asthma tripled in the late 20th century in a mysterious trend often called the "allergy epidemic."

Today, one in five American children have a respiratory allergy like hay fever, and nearly one in ten have asthma. Five percent of children are allergic to peanuts, milk and other foods, half again as many as fifteen years ago.

What's going on?

Again we look to the Amish for answers. On the basis of skin-prick tests, a mere 7.2 percent of the 138 Amish children tested by Dr. Mark Holbreich, an allergist in Indianapolis, were sensitized to tree pollens and other allergens. Those results made Indiana Amish among the *least* allergic populations ever described in the developed world. How is this possible? Scientists say it could be "the farm effect." On working farm, beginning as infants children are exposed to a huge variety of microorganisms: pollen, bacteria, dust, mold, insects—you name it, and it's either squishing underfoot, floating through the air, or under your fingernails. Dr. Holbreich said, "You do this every day for thirty years, 365 days a year, you can see there are so many exposures." Farms with the greatest array of microbes, including fungi, appear to be the most protective against asthma. And perhaps most amazingly, the benefits of farm life begin in utero. When a pregnant woman lives on a farm and is exposed to all the usual farm microbes, her child will have fewer allergies.

Getting out in nature isn't just psychologically uplifting—it's also good for your body!

You can also mix in gratitude as a way to feel better. What are you grateful for? This is a question you can always ask, and especially when you are walking. I do this.

Another way to empower yourself is to follow your breath as you walk. Notice your breathing. This helps bring you into the present moment. You can relieve pain and suffering. You can experience peace and tranquility. As you breathe in, notice it is your in-breath. As you breathe out, notice it is your out-breath. Pay attention to your breathing. This helps you get out of your mind and thoughts and reconnect with life.

Take one peaceful step. That is what Thich Nhat Hanh, the global spiritual leader, poet and peace activist, says. Notice your steps as you take them. This can be a walking meditation. You can feel comfortable.

Conclusion

In this book we've talked about the low-level laser as a healthy way to relieve pain and heal, and about avoiding opiates and non-steroidal anti-inflammatory drugs. We've discussed additional ways to be more comfortable and active.

Make sure you take action on what you have discovered in these chapters. I'll leave you with a secret for living an active and healthy life.

The secret is to do things constantly that are good for your well-being. Eat healthy food at each meal. Get some exercise. Laugh, meditate, and do breathing exercises throughout the day. Make sure your career is something you are content with. And when you have any pain, get low-level laser treatments so that you can be comfortable and heal.

Everything works synergistically—food, water, exercise, supplements, laser, relaxing exercises, laughter, breathing exercises, meditation, and gratitude. If you do most of these every day, you can have a wonderful life. Except laser, I do all of them daily. It is powerful if you do it all, but just doing one thing can help.

You can optimize your health. You can do the best you can with your current situation. You can eat healthily. You can make sure you are getting enough water. You can take some targeted nutritional supplement for your situation. You can do some relaxing exercises.

You can mix laughter in throughout each day. You can do breathing exercises during the day, even if you take just five minutes to do it. You can meditate. Again, maybe you meditate for half an hour, or maybe you meditate for just five minutes. You can get low-level laser treatments as needed. This will all help you be healthy. You will have energy. You will be doing the best you can. You will feel peaceful and relaxed every day. Your enjoyment of life will increase.

If you would like to move forward to discuss additional resources and ideas with me, call me at 520-363-1603 and leave your name and number, and I'll call you back.

Thank you—and may you always enjoy good health!